Adrenal 1

Balancing Your Hormones And Boosting Your Energy (Adrenal Reset, Anxiety Solution, Stress Management, Mind and Mood)

Sherry S. Williams

Insulin Resistance Diet: Secrets Revealed To Prevent Diabetes and Lose Weight (Optimize Your Body, Lose The Belly, Improve Hormones, Reverse Insulin Resistance)

This book was self-published with the amazing help of Self-Publishing Made Easy Now! [1] . You can grab a free copy of the checklist that started my journey here: FREE Self-Publishing Checklist [2] .

[1] https://selfpublishingmadeeasynow.com/xpjv
[2] https://selfpublishingmadeeasynow.com/free_checklist

Table of Contents

1 - Causes and Symptoms of Adrenal Fatigue

Adrenal fatigue is a term used to describe the signs and symptoms resulting from the failure of the adrenal glands to function optimally. A syndrome usually linked to prolonged or intense stress, adrenal fatigue may also result (during or after) from an acute or chronic infection such as influenza, pneumonia, bronchitis, and other respiratory infections.

The primary symptom of adrenal fatigue is fatigue that does not seem to go away after sleeping it off. The problem is that this condition is unlike other health conditions, such as ankle sprain, that you can easily pinpoint. You can suffer from adrenal fatigue and still appear and act like everything is all right in the world.

What the world cannot see is that under that seemingly normal exterior is a sense of tiredness and general un-wellness. It is common for individuals with adrenal fatigue to require stimulants like coffee and colas to get themselves going in the daytime.

What Your Adrenal Glands Do

What do your adrenal glands do for you? You have two of them, each one located above each of your kidneys. Your adrenal glands' cortex (outer section) is responsible for producing the hormones aldosterone and cortisol, while its inner section, the adrenal medulla, secretes the hormones norepinephrine and adrenaline.

The hormones cortisol, adrenaline, aldosterone, and norepinephrine perform several functions that include:

- Metabolism maintenance tasks like making sure your inflammation as well as blood sugar levels are stable

- Water-salt balance regulation by way of glucocorticoids and mineralocorticoids

- Control of your body's fight-or-flight defense mechanism during times of stress

- Providing the signal for beginning the body's sexual maturation as well as controlling its progress onward to puberty

- Pregnancy maintenance

Adrenal Fatigue Symptoms

You will know if you are suffering from adrenal fatigue by the presence of these symptoms:

- Unexplained tiredness that usually occurs early in the morning and in the middle of the afternoon

- Difficulty with getting out of bed in the morning, even if you have had a full sleep the night before

- Feeling overwhelmed, run down, or "gray"

- Having trouble in recovering from an illness or stressful experience

- Cravings for sweet and/or salty snack foods

- Feeling more alert and energetic after six o' clock in the evening than you do the entire day

Adrenal Fatigue Causes

As mentioned earlier, adrenal fatigue sets in when the adrenal glands fail to sufficiently manage stress. Your adrenal glands are responsible for mobilizing your response to physical, psychological, or emotional stress, and they do these by producing hormones that regulate various stress-coping mechanisms such as production and storage of energy, heart rate, immune function, and muscle tone.

It does not matter if the stress comes from a single minor spat or a series of major surgeries – your adrenal glands have to answer to the call of maintaining homeostasis in your system. They can get too stimulated from one intense stress or cumulative stresses, and as a result diminish their ability to produce the needed hormones. This causes them to respond insufficiently, giving way to adrenal fatigue.

To put it simply, adrenal fatigue generally stems from any of these stress factors:

- Poor nutrition, injury, surgery, exhaustion, addiction, and other sources of physical stress

- Relationship problems, crisis at work, and other unavoidable situations that trigger emotional or psychological stress

- Severe infection, recurrent illness, and other diseased states

- Severe/continuous environmental stress brought on by pollutants and toxic chemicals

2 - A Diet Plan to Defend Yourself against Adrenal Fatigue

What you put in your mouth is your primary weapon in overcoming adrenal fatigue. Follow these guidelines in supporting the health of your adrenal gland:

Eat at the proper times.

For people who suffer from adrenal fatigue, eating breakfast has to be prioritized. While you sleep, your body is actually fasting. Your body needs fuel that will help it last through the morning hours. This is the reason it is extremely important that you consume a protein source (high quality) as well as carbohydrates (complex) in small quantities.

You must also realize that having adrenal fatigue makes you likely to find it difficult to keep your blood sugar levels stable all through the day (since the hormone cortisol plays a key role in blood sugar stability). For this reason, you must focus on eating plenty of small meals all day to help your body avoid stresses, blood sugar crashes, and food cravings.

Have more fats and proteins.

A great way of giving your energy levels a sustained high without the dreaded blood sugar spikes is to make sure you are getting enough protein into your body. Go for healthy options such as wild fish, free-range chicken, beef, eggs, and protein powders (good quality). It helps if you try buying your meat organic; to save money, get them at the local farmers market.

When it comes to fats, choose to eat the healthy kinds, including coconut, cheese, avocado, butter, seeds and nuts. Getting adequate amounts of fat is important since they are great energy sources, as long as they come from wholly natural foods.

Eliminate caffeine from your diet.

Consuming caffeinated beverages may seem like a good idea, as they do make you feel temporarily energetic. The problem is that they add significant stress to the adrenal glands as well as the endocrine system. The caffeine contained in these drinks gear your adrenals into action, by secreting cortisol and adrenaline in the exact same way as they release these hormones during fight-or-flight responses.

Your adrenal glands eventually become depleted and less able to perform its normal functions. Individuals who suffer from adrenal fatigue often point out that coffee does not have any effect on them, but this is because their adrenal glands have already been through so much stimulation that it fails to respond effectively in times of stress.

Recognize your intolerances to certain foods.

Otherwise, your intolerance, sensitivity, and allergy to food will keep your gut from effectively digesting and excreting anything you take in. This is exactly why the first sign of food intolerance is constipation, diarrhea, and other problems with the digestive system.

Food intolerances also keep your body from fully digesting all those nutrients that your foods provide, which then leaves you running low on energy and feeling weakened. The same food issues also encourage gut inflammation, causing histamine to be released and causing you to sneeze and cough.

Because your food is not properly digested, unhealthy bacteria are allowed to flourish in your gut, which causes your immune system to become weakened.

3 - Adrenal Fatigue Diet Power Foods

Aside from the foods mentioned earlier, there are other adrenal fatigue diet approved foods you need to start stocking up on, such as the following:

Seaweed

Kelp, wakame, nori, and other types of seaweed are rich sources of different kinds of vitamins and minerals, one of which is magnesium; a cup of seaweed contains 218 milligrams. Your body needs magnesium to carry out more than three hundred processes, and it also helps relax your body, muscles, and mind.

You can easily incorporate seaweed into your diet by preparing rice rolls or veggie sushi rolls. Nori sheets are also great alternatives to wraps. Slice up small sections of wakame or kelp, then add to your stir-fries, stews, soups, and other dishes.

Himalayan/Celtic Salt

Your adrenal glands help in maintaining your body's mineral balance, which may be the reason a little more salt is good for them. Adding back essential minerals to your system with Himalayan salt or Celtic salt (steer clear of table salt) is a healthy way of giving your energy levels a boost. You can try mixing a bit of Himalayan/Celtic salt to your drinking water in the daytime for some overall energy increase.

Lemon

A lot of people suffering from adrenal fatigue actually have a highly acidic system, which is why consuming lemons is beneficial for them. Lemon can help balance the pH levels in your body, making it more alkaline and neutral and therefore less likely to experience inflammation. Increased inflammation in the body may be one cause of some of your adrenal fatigue symptoms.

Now, you would think that using lemon to alkaline your body sounds strange, especially since it is an acidic fruit. The great news is that once lemon is ingested, it becomes alkaline inside your body. You can start alkalizing your body by adding one tablespoon of freshly squeezed lemon juice to your warm water (one glass) in the morning. A pinch of Celtic or Himalayan salt would be a great finishing touch.

Mackerel and herring

phosphatidylserine is a natural substance (phospholipid) in the body that plays an important role in helping the brain's hypothalamus regulate adrenal/hormonal function as well as improving brain function, improving memory, and sharpening mental focus, and you can get it by eating fish like mackerel and herring.

Three and a half ounces of mackerel will provide you 480 milligrams of this lipid, while the same amount of herring should give you 350 milligrams. You may enjoy the health benefits of phosphatidylserine in both fresh and canned versions of mackerel and herring.

Peppers

Peppers are abundant in vitamin C, which is among the chief vitamins hosted by your adrenal glands. Whenever your body is under stress, it uses up vitamin C at a higher rate. This is why you must take in more vitamin C to promote adrenal health as well as help decrease your cortisol, which is your primary stress hormone.

Consider having pepper slices as your snack; you may also add them to salad dishes for a spicy kick and some energy boost. Keep in mind that peppers pack in more vitamin C power if you eat them raw.

Protein

You can help your body build more energy by eating protein from good quality sources. Protein contains B vitamins that are needed to produce energy and build your cells as well as promote fat metabolism, neurotransmitter synthesis, and nerve cell maintenance.

Your body also needs B vitamins to support your adrenals in times of stress. Go for whole protein sources such as liver, nuts, poultry, chicken, shellfish, fish, eggs, and meats. Make sure your every meal includes a portion of protein to provide your body long-lasting energy.

Eat your fat

Your body actually needs fat to synthesize hormones, many of which are produced by your adrenal glands. In fact, the adrenals are responsible for producing about fifty kinds of hormones. This is why a bit of additional healthy fat is good for you. Try using olive oil, walnut oil, flax seed oil, and coconut oil as well as butter and avocado on a more regular basis.

You may cook with them (coconut oil), drizzle them on dishes (olive oil), or use them in preparing homemade dressings (olive oil and flaxseed oil). It also helps to consume fish like tuna and salmon, both of which are rich sources of omega 3 fatty acids. Omega-3s can help reduce inflammation in your body and counteract the effects of adrenal fatigue.

4 - Pointers in Following the Adrenal Fatigue Diet Plan

Dietary Goals

- See to it that thirty to forty percent of your diet consists of vegetables. It is also important that ½ of your veggies are eaten raw.

- You should also keep in mind that twenty to thirty percent of your diet should be from animal sources, while another twenty to thirty percent has to come from healthy fats (including nuts and seeds).

- Make sure that whole grains comprise ten to twenty percent of your diet. Another ten to twenty percent has to come from legumes and beans, and the remaining ten to fifteen percent of your diet should be made of whole fruits.

- Your meals should be eaten frequently, and in small portions. The best time to have breakfast is between six and eight in the morning. Have your lunch at 12 noon, and your snacks at 10 a.m., 3 p.m., and an hour before bedtime.

- Avoid these foods at all costs: sugary snacks, white bread and other refined grains, processed foods, fast food, coffee, high sugar fruits, and dried fruits.

Diet Tricks

- Skipping breakfast as a diet trick should be ditched. You need to eat in the morning so that your blood sugar and energy levels are up.

- Avoid getting too hungry. You can do this by eating an early lunch, since your body can quickly use up the energy provided by your breakfast. To avoid this dilemma, you may also have a good snack in the middle of the morning. Otherwise, your body starts getting out of hand and produces too much cortisol. It is also best to eat your breakfast right away (within one hour of waking) so that you avoid getting your cortisol levels pumped up.

- Avoid overeating, which only places extra burden on every part of your digestive system as well as your adrenal glands.

- Begin your day with an alkalizing detox drink that consists of warm water and lemon juice (a tablespoon), apple cider vinegar (a capful), and Celtic/Himalayan salt (1/4 teaspoon). Your adrenal glands will find this beverage soothing.

- Make sure that each of your meals have a carbohydrate + a protein + a fat = a balanced approach to food + more sustained energy. If you have to add beans and legumes or whole grains to the equation, make sure to restrict your consumption to one cup daily. And don't forget to load up on those veggies - your body needs them for the vitamins and minerals they provide. Just keep in mind that some vegetables are also carbohydrates; use them to replace other carb options for a healthier meal and bigger nutrient load.

- If you need to have a snack before bedtime, make sure to eat it an hour before going to bed. Great evening snack options include a piece of fresh fruits smeared with a tablespoon of yogurt or nut butter, a slice of sweet potato or cheese, or a small handful of cooked chicken strips dipped in mashed avocado.

Practice To Keep Away From

- Eating dried fruits or whole fruits, or drinking fruit

juices, in the mornings: High amounts of fructose are contained in fruits, which when consumed can cause your blood sugar levels to increase and making your body fatigued the whole morning. Plenty of fruits also contain a large amount of potassium that can tip the sodium-potassium balance.

- Consuming white rice, bread and other baked goods, pasta, and other refined carbohydrates: These foods contain high amounts of sugars and refined carbo-hydrates that increase your blood sugar, after which the increased blood sugar level suddenly drops and causes the body to experience symptoms of hypogly-cemia.

- Enjoying fried foods, deep-fried foods, and foods con-taining hydrogenated oils: They all contain trans fats that change chemically when heated, and cause stress to your body.

- Eating bananas, oranges, grapefruits, and dried fruits like dried figs, dates, and raisins: They all contain high amounts of potassium that worsen the sodium-potassium balance brought on by adrenal fatigue.

- Consuming coffee, caffeinated teas, hot chocolate,

soft drinks, and candies: Not only do they contain high amounts of sugar, they also contain stimulants like caffeine that force your body to function beyond its normal pace, resulting in an adrenal crash.

- Using sugar, syrups, honey, and other sweeteners: They are loaded with too much sugar that can trigger a metabolic response that results in sudden dipping of blood sugar levels.

- Becoming addicted to allergenic foods or alcoholic drinks: They only bring on stress to your body.

- Eating your meals in a hurry: Rushing through your food puts a burden on your body's digestive system to work harder.

Practices To Live Out In Moderation

- Eating whole grains and unrefined grains: They do not cause your blood sugar levels to suddenly increase in the way that unrefined grains do. Plus, the nutrients they carry are greater compared to the calories they contain. It is best not to eat whole grains or unrefined grains during your breakfast though. This is the time when your body craves calories the most, so you may need to avoid them altogether.

- Eating whole fruits like mango, apples, grapes (some varieties), pears, papaya, kiwis, cherries, and plums: These fruits are rich sources of a number of phytonutrients – as well as high concentrations of sugar (better avoid eating them for breakfast).

- Using peanut oil, safflower oil, corn oil, sunflower oil, and other polyunsaturated fats: These types of oils are good sources of essential fatty acids, but they get converted into unhealthy fats when heated. Steer clear of these oils when cooking; you can drizzle them on cooked dishes instead.

Practices To Commit To

- Eating your first meal of the day before ten in the morning: Your body will be more stable and healthy if it gets replenished right away (a whole night of sleeping = low glycogen reserves).

- Making sure your every meal has a wide array of protein, whole grains, and fats: Getting your energy from multiple sources ensures that your body has access to quick-release energy (whole grains), medium release energy (fats), and long term energy (protein).

- Combining different protein sources (legume, fish, fowl, animal, and dairy): Doing it this way assures you of a more balanced nutrition and sustainable energy.

- Getting six to eight servings of different kinds of vegetables, especially the brightly colored ones: These are rich sources of antioxidants, vitamins, minerals, and phytonutrients.

- Eating multiple meals and snacks the whole day: Eating this way allows your body to get a boost of energy all through the day, as your blood sugar is kept stable (and spikes/crashes are prevented).

- Consuming vegetable sprouts and baby veggies: They contain extremely high levels of nutrients.

- Using monounsaturated fats and oils: You can use them in low-heat cooking; just make sure to splash the pan with water before adding in the oil (this keeps it from overheating).

- Eating fresh, raw, soaked seeds and nuts: Eating

them in this manner allows your body to digest them more easily and makes their nutrients more available for your body to use.

5 - Recipes For Breakfast

Instead of starting every day with a glass of orange juice concentrate and a bowl of sugar-laden cereal, load up on these breakfasts that give your energy levels that much needed boost.

Veggies and Salmon Frittata

Ingredients:

- Eggs (6 pieces)

- Asparagus, chopped (1 bunch)

- Salt, kosher (1/2 teaspoon)

- Pepper, freshly cracked (1/2 teaspoon)

- Parsley, fresh, chopped (1 tablespoon)

- Cheese, grated (1/2 cup)

- Zucchini, sliced into quarters (1 piece)

- Salmon, tinned, drained (14 ½ ounces)

- Milk (1/4 cup)

- Coconut oil, for cooking

Directions:

1. Preheat the grill.

2. Heat a large skillet on medium-high before adding the oil. Add the onions and sauté for five minutes or until browned.

3. Stir in the asparagus and zucchini. Cook for two minutes or until tender and crunchy.

4. Meanwhile, place the eggs in a bowl. Pour in the milk, then beat well. Add the salt, pepper, and parsley; mix well.

5. Once the vegetables are done, stir in the salmon, making sure to break it up into pieces.

6. Add the egg mixture on top of the skillet contents, making sure to tilt the pan so that they are evenly covered with the eggs.

7. Reduce heat to medium-low and allow the entire mixture to cook for about three to five minutes.

8. Once the top appears to be cooked, sprinkle on the

cheese. Cook the surface as well as brown the cheese by placing under the grill.

9. Once done, transfer onto a large plate, slice, and serve.

Coconut Amaranth with Almond Flakes

Ingredients:

- Coconut, desiccated/flaked (1/8 cup)

- Coconut milk (1/3 cup)

- Stevia (1/2 teaspoon)

- Cinnamon (1/2 teaspoon)

- Strawberries, fresh (1/4 cup)

- Raspberries, fresh (1/4 cup)

- Water (1 cup)

- Amaranth (1/2 cup)

- Vanilla bean paste (1 teaspoon)

- Almonds, flaked (1 tablespoon)

Directions:

1. Pour the coconut milk and water into a large saucepan.

2. Add the amaranth and stir well to combine.

3. Heat on medium. Allow the mixture to boil before reducing heat to low.

4. Simmer for about twenty to twenty-five minutes or until all liquid is absorbed.

5. Add the vanilla bean paste, cinnamon, and coconut. Stir to combine.

6. Serve topped with berries and almond flakes.

7. Enjoy.

Almond Buckwheat Crepes

Ingredients:

- Salt, kosher (1/2 teaspoon)

- Coconut oil, melted (1/2 cup + 1 tablespoon)

- Greek yogurt, plain, nonfat (1/2 cup)

- Water (1/2 cup)

- Plums, ripe (6 to 8 pieces)

- Almonds, flaked (1/4 cup)

- Buckwheat flour (1 ¼ cups)

- Eggs, large (3 pieces)

- Almond milk (1 cup)

Directions:

1. Place the flour in a large bowl. Stir with the salt and set aside.

2. Place the eggs in another bowl. Add the milk, water, and oil. Stir well to combine.

3. Pour the egg mixture into the flour mixture. Stir until everything is well-combined and smooth.

4. Meanwhile, heat a large skillet on medium. Add coconut oil (1 tablespoon); once heated, pour in some of the prepared crepe mixture (it should be just enough to form a thin layer over the entire pan.

5. Cook for about one to two minutes or until the surface is no longer wet and the bottom is mostly browned. Flip to cook on the other side for another one to two minutes. Do the same with the rest of the batter.

6. Once done, serve the crepes topped with Greek yogurt, chopped plums, and flaked almonds.

7. Enjoy.

Spinach Egg Muffins

Ingredients:

- Baby spinach, packed, chopped roughly (1 ½ cups)

- Milk, cow's/almond/coconut (a splash)

- Eggs (4 to 5 pieces)

- Sea salt (a pinch)

- Pepper, freshly cracked (a pinch)

- Onion, large, diced (1/2 piece)

- Cherry tomatoes, halved (8 pieces)

Directions:

1. Set the oven at 360 degrees.

2. Use olive oil to lightly coat 4 muffin cups. Set aside.

3. Meanwhile, heat a skillet (non-stick) on medium-low. Add the oil and onions, ten sauté for about five minutes or until browned.

4. Remove the pan from the heat. Stir in the spinach and mix with onions. Continue stirring until the spinach is wilted.

5. Once done, transfer the mixture into the greased muffin cups. Top each muffin cup mixture with four halved tomatoes. Set aside.

6. Place the eggs in a medium bowl. Add the salt, pepper, and milk. Whisk well to combine, then pour on top of the tomato-topped muffin cups.

7. Place in the oven to bake for about twenty minutes or until the top is browned and puffy.

8. Remove from the oven once the spinach egg muffins are done. Let cool for several minutes.

9. Serve and enjoy.

Coco-Berry Pancakes

Ingredients:

- Coconut flour (1/3 cup)

- Eggs, medium (4 pieces)

- Blueberries, fresh (1/4 cup)

- Almond milk, unsweetened (1 tablespoon)

- Vanilla extract, pure (1 teaspoon)

- Bananas, large, ripe (2 pieces)

- Coconut oil – to be used in frying

Directions:

1. Fill a blender or food processor with the almond milk and eggs.

2. Add the coconut flour, vanilla extract, and bananas.

3. Process until the mixture is well-combined and smooth.

4. Meanwhile, heat a large pan (non-stick) on medium before adding the coconut oil (1/2 teaspoon).

5. Add the pancake mixture (two to three dollops at a time) and spread evenly by tilting the pan. Cook for about two to three minutes or until starting to bubble on the surface. Flip to cook on the other side for two minutes more or until golden brown.

6. Serve and enjoy.

6 - Recipes For Lunch

Eat these healthy lunches to help your body recover from adrenal fatigue.

Sweet Potato Curry

Ingredients:

- Baby corn (1 cup)

- Onion, medium brown, chopped finely (1 piece)

- Bell pepper, red, diced (1 piece)

- Vegetable stock (1 cup)

- Cilantro, fresh, chopped finely (a large handful)

- Curry paste, red Thai (2 tablespoons)

- Bell pepper, green, diced (1 piece)

- Sweet potato, large, peeled, chopped into half-inch cubes (2 pieces)

- Cashew nuts (a small handful)

- Coconut oil (1 teaspoon)

- Coconut milk (16 ounces)

- Snow peas (1 cup)

- Red chili, chopped finely (1 piece)

Directions:

1. Heat a large skillet on medium. Add the oil.

2. Once the oil is heated, add the onion. Stir and cook for about three to four minutes or until softened but not browned.

3. Add the curry paste. Stir and cook for about one minute before adding the coconut milk.

4. Pour in the sweet potatoes and vegetable stock as well. Stir again, cover the pan, and allow the mixture to cook for about ten to fifteen minutes.

5. Once the potatoes are slightly tenderized, add the snow peas, baby corn, and peppers. Stir and cook uncovered for another ten to fifteen minutes or until all veggies are cooked through.

6. Transfer the cooked curry onto a platter. Add cashew nuts, cilantro, and chili on top.

7. Serve immediately.

Tasty Quinoa Meatloaf

Ingredients:

- Garlic cloves (2 pieces)

- Sea salt (1/4 teaspoon)

- Pepper, freshly cracked (1/4 teaspoon)

- Eggs (2 pieces)

- Basil, dried (1/2 teaspoon)

- Olive oil, extra virgin (1 tablespoon)

- Chili powder (1/2 teaspoon)

- Beef mince, regular (1/2 pound)

- Beef liver (1/2 pound)

- Tomatoes, chopped (14 ounces)

- Onion, brown, chopped finely (1 piece)

- Quinoa (1/3 cup)

- Thyme (1/2 teaspoon)

- Oregano (1/2 teaspoon)

- Oregano, dried (1/2 teaspoon)

Directions:

1. Follow package directions in cooking the quinoa. Set aside in a large bowl.

2. Meanwhile, heat a medium non-stick skillet on medium. Add the onion and cook for about three to four minutes or until translucent and softened.

3. Add the garlic. Stir and cook for about one to two minutes or until tender and fragrant.

4. Set the oven at 350 degrees to preheat.

5. Add the cooked garlic and onion (1/2 portion) to the bowl containing the cooked quinoa. Add the herbs, salt, pepper, mince, and eggs. Stir until evenly combined.

6. Meanwhile, use baking paper to line a loaf tin (1-pound). Pour in the mince mixture and press well to make sure the loaf tin is evenly covered.

7. Place in the oven to bake for about forty to forty-five minutes or until completely cooked. Cover with foil once the meat mixture starts browning too quickly

8. In the meantime, heat a large non-stick pan on medium. Add the basil, oregano, the remaining cooked onion, and tomatoes. Stir and cook for about fifteen minutes or until well-mixed.

9. Once the quinoa meatloaf is done, remove from the oven and let on a cooling rack. After five minutes, transfer onto a large plate.

10. Serve topped with fresh parsley bits and enjoy.

Chicken Broccoli Salad with Honey-Mustard Dressing

Ingredients:

- Broccoli, small, chopped into florets (3 pieces)

- Coconut oil (3 teaspoons)

- Chicken breast, sliced thinly (500 grams)

- Onion, red, finely sliced (1 piece)

- Dressing:

- Thyme, dried (1/2 teaspoon)

- Lemon juice, freshly squeezed (1 tablespoon)

- Honey (1 tablespoon)

- Garlic oil (1/2 teaspoon) or garlic, minced (1/2 teaspoon)

- Mustard, whole grain (1 teaspoon)

- Tamari sauce (1 tablespoon)

Directions:

1. Place all the ingredients for the dressing in a medium bowl. Stir well to combine and set aside half of the mixture.

2. Meanwhile, pour the other half of the dressing into a large bowl. Add the chicken strips and let sit to marinate.

3. Fill steaming pot with the broccoli and chicken strips. Cook for about five minutes or until just cooked.

4. Meanwhile, heat a non-stick skillet on medium-high before adding the coconut oil (1 teaspoon). Stir in the onions and cook until browned nicely. Place in a small bowl and set aside.

5. Pour in more coconut oil (2 teaspoons) to the same skillet. Allow the oil to melt before adding in the steamed chicken.

6. Cook the chicken for five minutes or until evenly browned on all sides. Make sure the chicken strips are not nice and tender, not overcooked.

7. Remove from heat and let the cooked chicken sit for about two minutes or until completely cooked.

8. Reheat the skillet and add the sliced red onions, the rest of the dressing, and the steamed broccoli. Stir until all ingredients are mixed.

9. Cook for one minute or until the entire mixture is heated through.

10. Serve right away.

Kale Omelet

Ingredients:

- Cauliflower, chopped (1 cup)

- Milk (a splash)

- Kale, large bushy leaf, finely chopped (1 piece)

- Onion, sliced (1/2 piece)

- Zucchini, sliced into halves then strips (1/2 piece)

- Pepper, freshly cracked (1/4 teaspoon)

- Tomato, diced (1 piece)

- Bell pepper, red (1/2 piece)

- Eggs (6 pieces)

- Coconut oil, for cooking

Directions:

1. Heat a large skillet (non-stick) before adding in the oil. Stir in the onions and cauliflower. Once the onions are browned and the cauliflower is almost

cooked through.

2. Stir in the chopped kale, zucchini strips, and diced to-mato. Turn heat down to medium-low and allow the mixture to cook for several minutes.

3. Meanwhile, place the eggs in a medium bowl. Add the milk and pepper, then whisk until combined.

4. Heat another non-stick skillet on medium. Add the oil; once heated, pour in the egg mixture and cook for several minutes or until about set.

5. Flip the omelet on the other side with a spatula to cook for a few minutes.

6. Once done, slice the omelet in half and transfer onto 2 individual plates.

7. Add the veggie mixture on top of each omelet slice.

8. Serve and enjoy.

Baby Spinach Salad with Salmon Cakes

Ingredients:

- Spring onion, sliced (1 piece)

- Cherry tomatoes (12 pieces)

- Sea salt (1/4 teaspoon)

- Pepper, freshly cracked (1/4 teaspoon)

- Balsamic vinegar (2 tablespoons)

- Almond flour/meal (1/2 cup)

- Coconut oil, for cooking

- Salmon, tinned (14 ½ ounces)

- Parsley, fresh, chopped (2 tablespoons)

- Egg (1 piece)

- Baby spinach (4 cups)

- Olives (12 pieces)

- Olive oil, extra virgin (2 tablespoons)

Directions:

1. Drain the salmon and place in a large bowl.

2. Add the parsley and onion as well as pepper and salt.

3. Stir to combine and make sure the salmon is evenly coated, before breaking up with a fork. Give the mixture a good stir, then crack in the egg.

4. Stir all ingredients until well-combined. Set aside.

5. Meanwhile, pour the almond meal onto a large plate. Place another clean plate beside it.

6. Mold the salmon mixture into 4 balls before patting them down into patties. Coat each patty with the almond meal and place on the clean plate.

7. Heat a large skillet (non-stick) on medium. Add the oil; once heated, add the patties. Turn heat down to low and cook each patty for about five minutes on all sides or until nicely browned and cooked through.

8. Rinse the spinach and place on 2 plates. Slice the cherry tomatoes into halves and place next to the spinach to form a salad bed.

9. Pour the balsamic vinegar and olive oil in a small bowl. Stir well to combine before drizzling ½ of the mixture over the salad.

10. Top each salad with 2 salmon cakes. Drizzle with the

remaining dressing and serve.

7 - Recipes For Dinner

Eating these adrenal fatigue diet dinners before six in the evening can help in replenishing your body's energy stores.

Easy Liver Skewers

Ingredients:

- Green pepper (1 piece)

- Red pepper (1 piece)

- Paprika, smoked (1/2 teaspoon)

- Green apple (1 piece)

- Sea salt (a pinch)

- Pepper, freshly cracked (a pinch)

- Chicken livers, chopped into one-inch cubes (3/4 pound)

- Lettuce leaves

Directions:

1. Place the chopped chicken livers in a large bowl.

2. Chop the peppers and apple into one-inch cubes, then add to the chicken liver cubes.

3. Thread the cubed pieces onto skewers (6 to 8 pieces), making sure to alternate (liver, pepper, apple).

4. Use a bit of olive oil to lightly coat the pieces, then season with pepper, paprika, and salt.

5. Grill for about ten minutes or until the liver is cooked through (make sure to turn the skewers frequently).

6. Serve on a bed of lettuce leaves and enjoy.

Apple and Chicken Liver Salad

Ingredients:

- Spinach leaves (1 cup)

- Onion, large, white (1 piece)

- Hazelnuts (1/2 cup)

- Chicken livers, cut into one-inch cubes (3/4 pound)

- Rocket leaves (1 cup)

- Blueberries, fresh (1/2 cup)

- Apple, green, sliced into cubes (1 piece)

- Olive oil, extra virgin (1 tablespoon)

Dressing:

- Honey (2 tablespoons)

- Garlic cloves, crushed (1 piece)

- Salt, kosher (1/4 teaspoon)

- Pepper, freshly cracked (1/4 teaspoon)

- Lemon juice, freshly squeezed (1/4 cup)

- Thyme, fresh, chopped (2 tablespoons)

- Olive oil, extra virgin (1/4 cup)

Directions:

1. Place the ingredients for the salad (save for the livers) in a large mixing bowl.

2. Heat a large skillet (non-stick) on medium before adding the coconut oil (1 tablespoon).

3. Stir in the chicken livers and cook until golden brown.

4. Combine the ingredients for the dressing.

5. Add the cooked chicken livers to the salad ingredients. Toss gently to combine.

6. Serve the salad topped with the prepared dressing.

Chicken Curry

Ingredients:

- Onion, diced (1 piece)

- Curry powder (1 teaspoon)

- Coconut cream (1/2 cup)

- Carrot, halved, sliced (1 piece)

- Chicken, diced (14 ounces)

- Turmeric powder (2 teaspoons)

- Coconut oil – to be used in cooking

- Brown rice/rice noodles, cooked

- Lettuce, shredded

Directions:

1. Heat a large skillet (non-stick) on high before adding the oil.

2. Stir in the onions and carrots; cook for three to four minutes or until the onions are browned and the carrots have tenderized.

3. Add the chicken to cook for about two minutes, before stirring in the turmeric and curry powder. Cook for an additional two minutes before stirring in the coconut cream.

4. Allow the mixture to simmer for about one to two minutes or until heated through. Remove from heat and let cool for about five minutes.

5. Pour over cooked brown rice or rice noodles. Top with shredded lettuce.

6. Serve and enjoy.

Stir-Fried Chicken Livers

Ingredients:

- Chicken livers, sliced into one-inch cubes (1 pound)

- Bell pepper, green, sliced into strips (1 piece)

- Ginger, fresh, grated, 1" (1 piece)

- Bean sprouts, fresh (1 cup)

- Red chilies, medium, sliced thinly (2 pieces)

- Spring onions (2 pieces)

- Coconut oil (2 tablespoons)

- White onion, large, sliced thinly (1 piece)

- Garlic cloves, crushed (2 pieces)

- Bell pepper, red, sliced into strips (1 piece)

- Snow peas (4 ounces)

- Coconut aminos (3 tablespoons)

- Water (1 tablespoon)

Directions:

1. Heat a large skillet (non-stick) on medium. Add the coconut oil, then the liver. Stir-fry for five minutes or until completely browned.

2. Transfer the cooked liver onto a large plate. Meanwhile, add onions to the skillet and cook for about two to three minutes or until slightly softened.

3. Stir in the garlic, chilis, and ginger. Cook for another two minutes before adding in the snow peas and peppers.

4. Once the snow peas and peppers are slightly softened, stir in the bean sprouts. Cook for one minute before adding the liver as well as water and coconut aminos.

5. Increase heat to high and cook for about two to three minutes or until heated through and evenly combined.

6. Serve immediately with chilis and spring onions on top. Enjoy.

Crockpot Beef Stew

Ingredients:

- Onion, diced (1 piece)

- Turmeric (2 teaspoons)

- Sweet paprika (1 tablespoon)

- Carrots, chopped into chunks (4 pieces)

- Cumin (1 teaspoon)

- Cauliflower, chopped into chunks (2 ½ cups)

- Gravy beef, diced (2 1/5 pounds)

- Tomatoes, diced (14 ounces)

- Thyme, dried (1/4 teaspoon)

- Chili flakes (1/4 teaspoon)

- Water/stock (1 cup)

Directions:

1. Fill the crock pot with all ingredients (save for the

cauliflower and carrots).

2. Stir to combine.

3. Cook on high for three hours.

4. Stir in the cauliflower and carrots. Cook for an additional three hours.

5. Serve and enjoy.

8 - Recipes For Snacks

Substitute your favorite coffee and sugary snacks with these healthy, adrenal fatigue diet approved snack recipes – long-lasting energy will be on its way.

Nori-Wrapped Tuna Salad

Ingredients:

- Carrot, grated (1 piece)

- Tuna, drained (6 ½ ounces)

- Fennel, fresh, chopped finely (1/4 piece)

- Sweet potato (1 piece)

- Nori seaweed (4 pieces)

- Avocado (1 piece)

- Tomato, sliced (1 piece)

- Lettuce, shredded

Directions:

1. Take a sheet of foil and top with the nori.

2. Place avocado on top of the nori.

3. Layer the rest of the ingredients.

4. Roll tightly.

5. Serve and enjoy.

Easy Roast Salad with Mediterranean Salad Dressing

Ingredients:

- Carrots, sliced lengthwise into quarters (4 to 5 pieces)

- Lettuce leaves, mixed (2 cups)

- Hot Cajun spice (1/2 teaspoon)

- Chicken drumsticks (5 to 6 pieces)

- Sweet potatoes, small (2 pieces)

- Olive oil

- Mediterranean salad dressing:

- Dijon mustard (2 teaspoons)

- Pepper, freshly cracked (1/2 teaspoon)

- Feta cheese, crumbled (1/2 cup)

- Oregano, dried (1 teaspoon)

- Vinegar, red wine (2 tablespoons)

- Kosher salt (1/2 teaspoon)

- Olive oil, extra virgin (1/2 cup)

- Parsley, fresh, chopped (1 tablespoon)

- Plum tomato, diced (1 piece)

Directions:

1. Set the oven at 420 degrees.

2. Arrange all the carrots, lettuce leaves, sweet potatoes, and chicken drumsticks on a large baking tray. Drizzle with the olive oil before sprinkling with the hot Cajun spice.

3. Make sure everything is well-coated, then place in the oven to bake for one hour or until tender.

4. Place all ingredients for the dressing in a medium bowl. Stir to combine; set aside.

5. Place the lettuce leaves on a platter. Add the other vegetables on top.

6. Pour on the dressing and serve immediately.

7. Sesame Coated Egg Nori Rolls

Ingredients:

- Coconut aminos (1 tablespoon)

- Chives, chopped finely (1/8 cup)

- Eggs, large (4 pieces)

- Nori sheets (2 to 4 pieces)

- Milk (2 tablespoons)

- Sesame oil (1/2 tablespoon)

- Chili flakes (1 teaspoon)

- Ginger, grated (1/2 teaspoon)

- Sesame seeds (2 tablespoons)

Directions:

1. Place the eggs in a large bowl. Add the chives, grated ginger, chili flakes, milk, and coconut aminos. Whisk until everything is well-combined.

2. Heat a medium size saucepan on medium before adding the sesame oil. Add the egg mixture (1 ladleful) and cook for about one to two minutes or until bubbling on the surface but not cooked through.

3. Once the pancakes are done, remove from the skillet and set on a large plate.

4. Top each pancake with a nori sheet, then roll tightly (make sure the nori is inside the roll). Do the same with the rest of the pancakes.

5. Slice each egg nori roll into one-inch portions. Place on a serving platter and coat with the sesame seeds.

6. Serve and enjoy.

Wakame Spinach Salad

Ingredients:

- Wakame, dried (1/2 cup)

- Cucumber (1/2 piece)

- Lemon juice, freshly squeezed (1 tablespoon)

- Baby spinach/rocket (2 cups)

- Avocado, ripe (1 piece)

- Sesame seeds (1 tablespoon)

- Salt, kosher (1/2 teaspoon)

- Pepper, freshly cracked (1/2 teaspoon)

- Water, lukewarm

Directions:

1. Place the wakame in a large bowl. Fill with enough lukewarm water to cover and add the cider vinegar (2 tablespoons). Let sit for about ten minutes or until the wakame is rehydrated (it should appear swelled and glossy).

2. Place spinach on a large plate. Set aside.

3. After draining the wakame, place on top of the spin-

ach. Add the cucumber and avocado.

4. Drizzle with lemon juice and sprinkle with salt, pepper, and sesame seeds.

5. Serve and enjoy.

Spicy Deviled Eggs

Ingredients:

- Rice vinegar (1/2 teaspoon)

- Yogurt, natural, full fat (2 tablespoons)

- Ginger, crushed (1/2 teaspoon)

- Chili powder, mild (1/4 teaspoon)

- Eggs (8 pieces)

- Wasabi (1/2 teaspoon)

- Nori sheet, chopped into 0.5 cm portions (1/2 piece)

- Spring onions, chopped finely (1 tablespoon)

Directions:

1. Pour cool water into a large saucepan. Add the eggs and heat on medium.

2. Once the water is boiling, turn off the heat. Cover and let sit for about ten minutes.

3. Take the eggs out and place in a bowl filled with iced water. After one minute, remove the eggshells.

4. Slice eggs into lengthwise halves before scooping out the egg yolks.

5. Place egg yolks in a large bowl. Add the wasabi along with the yogurt, ginger, rice vinegar, and nori. Mash together to combine.

6. Transfer the egg yolk mixture into a star-tipped piping bag. Squeeze to fill the egg white holes with the egg yolk mixture.

7. Serve your deviled eggs topped with spring onions and mild chilli.

9 - Recipes For Bone Broth

These bone broths are boiled, simmered, and cooked thoroughly to extract all the nutrients as well as healing compounds that your body needs to fight off adrenal fatigue.

Carrots and Chicken Bone Broth

Ingredients:

- Carrots, chopped (3 pieces)

- Apple cider vinegar (3 tablespoons)

- Onions, medium, unpeeled, sliced lengthwise into quarters (2 pieces)

- Parsley, fresh (5 to 6 sprigs)

- Himalayan salt (1 teaspoon)

- Water, cold (18 to 20 cups)

- Chicken wings/feet/neck (4 pounds)

- Celery, chopped (3 stalks)

- Garlic cloves, unpeeled, smashed (4 pieces)

- Peppercorns, whole (1 teaspoon)

- Bay leaves (2 pieces)

- Thyme, fresh (3 sprigs)

- Oregano (1 teaspoon)

Directions:

1. Fill a crock pot (10-quarts) with all the ingredients.

2. Cook on low for twenty-four to forty-eight hours, making sure to skim off fat occasionally.

3. Once done, remove from heat. Allow the bone broth to cool a bit before straining the solids through a colander into a large bowl.

4. Allow the bone broth to cool down to room temperature. Cover and place in the refrigerator to chill.

5. Enjoy within one week (or place in the freezer and use within three months).

Satisfying Pork Bone Broth

Ingredients:

- Water (8 cups)

- Carrot, medium, peeled, sliced into cubes (1 piece)

- Fish sauce (2 tablespoons)

- Leeks, medium, cleaned, sliced crosswise into halves (2 pieces)

- Pork bones (2 ½ pounds)

- Apple cider vinegar (1 teaspoon)

Directions:

- Fill the pressure cooker (6-quarts) with the vegetables. Add the bones and fill with water to 2/3 capacity.

- Stir in the fish sauce and vinegar before securing the pressure cooker lid.

- Cook on high for thirty minutes to two hours.

- Discard any scum, then strain the mixture into a serving bowl.

- Serve and enjoy.

Garlic and Beef Bone Broth

Ingredients:

- Beef/chicken bones (2 pounds)

- Carrots (2 pieces)

- Apple cider vinegar (2 tablespoons)

- Water, filtered (4 quarts)

- Garlic cloves, peeled, crushed (8 pieces)

- Celery stalks (2 pieces)

- Sea salt, Himalayan (1 tablespoon)

Directions:

1. Fill a large pot with the beef/chicken bones, crushed garlic, salt, celery, and carrots.

2. Pour in the filtered water and apple cider vinegar. Stir to combine and heat the pot on medium-high.

3. Allow the entire mixture to come to a boil before turning the heat down to low.

4. Simmer for about twelve to twenty-four hours.

5. Once done, remove from heat and allow to completely cool. Strain through a fine-mesh strainer into a large bowl.

6. Pour into food containers and store in the refrigerator for two to three days (or freeze and use within three months).

7. Reheat in the microwave before drinking or using in your cooking.

Turkey Bone Broth with Cabbage and Potatoes

Ingredients:

- Water (4 quarts)

- Salt, kosher (1 ½ teaspoons)

- Tomatoes, whole, peeled, chopped (28 ounces)

- Paprika (1/4 teaspoon)

- Celery stalks, diced (2 pieces)

- Basil, dried (1 teaspoon)

- Onion, large, diced (1 piece)

- Bay leaf (1 piece)

- Potatoes, small, diced (6 pieces)

- Parsley, dried (1 teaspoon)

- Cabbage, shredded (1 ½ cups)

- Turkey carcass (1 piece)

- Carrots, large, diced (4 pieces)

- Barley, uncooked (1/2 cup)

- Worcestershire sauce (1 tablespoon)

- Black pepper, freshly cracked (1/4 teaspoon)

- Poultry seasoning (1/4 teaspoon)

- Thyme, dried (1 pinch)

Directions:

1. Fill a large stock pot with water. Add the turkey car-

cass and heat on medium-high.

2. Allow the water to come to a boil; turn the heat down to a simmer.

3. Cook the carcass for one hour or until all the meat fall off the bones.

4. Take the carcass out. Remove the turkey meat as well and chop into pieces; place in a medium bowl.

5. Pour the broth into another stock pot through a strainer (fine mesh). Stir in the chopped turkey meat and heat on medium.

6. Allow the mixture to boil before reducing heat to low. Add the vegetables as well as the spices and seasonings.

7. Simmer the mixture for one more hour or until the veggies are tender.

8. Discard the bay leaf before transferring the bone broth into serving bowls.

9. Serve and enjoy.

Lamb Marrow Bone Broth

Ingredients:

- Water, filtered (8 cups)

- Bay leaf (1 piece)

- Lamb marrow bones (1 kilogram)

- Onion, peeled, quartered (1 piece)

- Celery stalks, chopped roughly (2 pieces)

- Sea salt, Celtic (1/4 teaspoon)

- Black pepper, freshly cracked (1/4 teaspoon)

- Coconut oil, extra virgin (60 milliliters)

- Carrots, peeled, chopped roughly (2 pieces)

- Garlic cloves (3 pieces)

- Apple cider vinegar (2 tablespoons)

Directions:

1. Set the oven at 400 degrees to preheat.

2. Heat a casserole dish (flame-proof) over medium heat. Add the coconut oil and allow to melt. Stir in the bones, cover the dish, and place in the oven.

3. Bake for about thirty minutes or until the lamb marrow bones are browned.

4. Remove the dish from the oven and place on the stovetop. Pour in the filtered water, seasonings, and the rest of the ingredients.

5. Allow the entire mixture to boil before reducing heat to low. Simmer for about four to six hours, adding more water as needed.

6. Turn off the heat. Allow the bone broth to cool before straining and placing in the refrigerator.

7. Remove the congealed fats from the chilled bone broth. Pour into an airtight jar and refrigerate, or pour into ice cube trays and freeze.

10 - Recipes For Fermented Foods

Abundant in probiotics and minerals, these fermented foods allow your body to properly digest food, effectively absorb nutrients, and bring your energy levels up.

Black Sesame Beet Salad

Ingredients:

- Olive oil, extra virgin, divided (3 tablespoons)

- Miso, white (1/4 cup)

- Watercress, trimmed (1 bunch)

- Vinegar, rice wine (2 tablespoons)

- Black sesame seeds (1 teaspoon) or white sesame seeds, toasted (1 teaspoon)

- Beets, small, golden, scrubbed, divided (6 pieces)

- Salt, kosher (1/4 teaspoon)

- Black pepper, freshly ground (1/4 teaspoon)

Directions:

1. Set the oven at 400 degrees.

2. Meanwhile, use foil to hold the beets (4 pieces). Pour on the oil (1 tablespoon) and rub on the beets until evenly coated.

3. Sprinkle the beets with pepper and salt before closing up the foil. Place inside a baking sheet (rimmed) and bake in the oven for about thirty to forty minutes or until tender and roasted through.

4. Remove the beets from the foil and let cool on a plate. Once cooled, peel off the skins and slice the flesh into half-inch wedges. Set aside.

5. Pour the vinegar into a medium bowl. Add the miso, water (3 tablespoons), and remaining oil (2 tablespoons). Whisk well to combine and set aside.

6. Slice the remaining beets (2 pieces) into thin cuts. Place on a platter along with the watercress and the roasted beets.

7. Pour on the prepared dressing before sprinkling the sesame seeds.

8. Serve and enjoy.

Bold Brussels Sprouts Kimchi

Ingredients:

- Brussels sprouts, small, trimmed, halved (1 ½ pounds)

- Sriracha sauce (2 tablespoons)

- Scallions, sliced (2 pieces)

- Soy sauce, reduced sodium (1 tablespoon)

- Red pepper powder, Korean, coarse (1/4 cup)

- Fennel seeds, crushed (2 teaspoons)

- Kosher salt (3 ½ ounces + 7/10 ounces)

- Onion, small, chopped coarsely (1/2 piece)

- Garlic cloves (4 pieces)

- Fish sauce (2 tablespoons)

- Ginger, peeled, grated (1 tablespoon)

- Coriander seeds, crushed (2 teaspoons)

Directions:

1. Fill a large bowl with warm water (2 quarts) and salt (3 ½ ounces). Whisk until the salt is completely dissolved.

2. Add the Brussels sprouts to the brine; cover with a large plate to keep the Brussels sprouts down. Set aside for four hours at room temperature.

3. Rinse the brine-soaked Brussels sprouts before draining and placing inside a large bowl. Set aside.

4. Meanwhile, fill a food processor with the scallions, gochugaru, sriracha, coriander, onion, garlic, fish sauce, soy sauce, and fennel seeds. Process until the mixture is evenly blended and smooth.

5. Pour the mixture on top of the Brussels sprouts. Toss gently to combine before transferring into 2 canning jars (32-ounces). Make sure to press down until packed and all air pockets are released.

6. Fill a large bowl with the rest of the warm water (1 quart) and salt (0.7 ounces). Whisk to dissolve the salt completely before adding to the jars, making sure leave an inch of headspace.

7. Cover and let sit at room temperature, away from direct sunlight, for about three to five days, or until the mixture develops a tangy taste and bubbles form when it is stirred.

8. Place in the refrigerator to chill, then serve and enjoy.

Sea Bass Marinated in Miso

Ingredients:

- Mirin sauce (2 tablespoons)

- Salt, kosher (1/4 teaspoon)

- Pepper, freshly ground (1/4 teaspoon)

- Sea bass, black, skin-on, w/ pin bones removed (12 ounces)

- Balsamic vinegar (1 tablespoon)

- Sugar (1/4 cup)

- Miso, white (2 tablespoons)

- Vegetable oil, divided (1 ½ tablespoons)

- Salad greens, mixed (4 kinds)

Directions:

1. Pour the miso, mirin, and sugar in a large bowl. Whisk well to combine.

2. Add the fish and turn until evenly coated with the prepared sauce. Cover and place in the refrigerator to chill for twelve to twenty-four hours.

3. Heat a medium skillet (non-stick) on medium before adding oil (1 tablespoon). Add the marinated fish (excluding the liquid) and sprinkle with pepper and salt. Cook for four minutes with the skin face-down or until caramelized; turn the fish over to cook on the other side for an additional three minutes.

4. In the meantime, heat another medium skillet (non-stick) on medium-high. Add the remaining oil (1/2 tablespoon) and greens; cook for one minute or until just wilted.

5. Season the greens with pepper and salt before transferring onto individual plates. Set aside.

6. Pour vinegar into the same skillet with which you

cooked the greens. Stir for thirty minutes or until the vinegar is thickened.

7. Add the reduced vinegar on top of the greens before placing the fish,

8. Serve and enjoy.

Kimchi Yogurt Fried Chicken

Ingredients:

- Vegetable oil (5 cups)

- Fish sauce, reduced sodium (1/3 cup)

- Chicken breasts, boneless, skin-on (2 pieces)

- Kosher salt (1 teaspoon)

- Cayenne pepper (1 teaspoon)

- Chicken thighs, boneless, skin-on (4 pieces)

- Chicken wings (2 pieces)

- Kimchi yogurt:

- Black peppercorns (1/2 teaspoon)

- Sesame oil, toasted (1 tablespoon)

- Hot sauce (2 cups)

- Chili powder (1/2 teaspoon)

- Coriander seeds, whole (1/2 teaspoon)

- Chicken bouillon, crushed (1/2 teaspoon)

- Greek yogurt, plain, nonfat (1/2 teaspoon)

- Cardamom (1 pod)

- Fennel seeds, whole (1/2 teaspoon)

- Fish sauce (2 tablespoons)

- Turmeric, ground (1/2 teaspoon)

- Garlic powder (1/2 teaspoon)

Directions:

1. Heat a small skillet on medium before adding the peppercorns, fennel seeds, coriander seeds, and cardamom pod. Toast for two minutes and set aside to cool.

2. Reserve the seeds from the cardamom pods and place in a spice mill. Grind the seeds and all other toasted spices, then place in a large bowl.

3. Add yogurt, sesame oil, garlic powder, chili powder, hot sauce, fish sauce, chicken bouillon, turmeric, and paprika to the toasted spices. Mix well and set aside in the refrigerator.

4. Fill another large bowl with the chicken. Add ½ of the chilled kimchi yogurt mixture and coat the chicken with it. Refrigerate for four hours to four days.

5. Meanwhile, heat a large skillet (cast iron) on medium-high; once the thermometer shows a temperature of 300 degrees, add the oil until one inch deep in the pan.

6. Place the rice flour (3/4 cup) in a large bowl. Add water (1 cup) and salt (1 teaspoon), then whisk until evenly combined and smooth.

7. Add the marinated chicken (minus the liquid) to the flour mixture. Turn to coat and fry for ten to twelve minutes or until cooked through and golden brown.

Once done, place on a wire rack and allow to cool.

8. Turn the heat up to 350 degrees. Meanwhile, combine the remaining rice flour (3/4 cup), water (3/4 cup), cayenne, and fish sauce. Add the fried chicken and turn to coat before frying again for six to eight minutes.

9. Serve chicken with the remaining kimchi yogurt mixture. Enjoy.

Tare and Miso Chicken Meatballs

Ingredients:

- Scallions, minced (1 cup)

- Sesame oil/canola oil (2 tablespoons + 1 tablespoon)

- Chicken, dark meat, ground, divided (2 pounds)

- Red miso (2 tablespoons)

- Basting sauce:

- Sugar, light brown, packed (3/4 teaspoon)

- Mirin (1/4 cup)

- Garlic clove, crushed (1 piece)

- Sake (2 tablespoons)

- Ginger, peeled, sliced (1/4 ounce)

- Chicken broth, low-salt (1/2 cup)

- Soy sauce, reduced sodium (1/4 cup)

- Black pepper, freshly ground (1/4 teaspoon)

- Scallion, chopped (1 piece)

Directions:

1. Heat a small skillet (non-stick) on medium before adding the ground chicken (1 ½ cups). Stir and cook for two minutes or until opaque and almost cooked through.

2. Place the cooked chicken on a large plate. Allow to cool before placing in a large bowl.

3. Add the rest of the chicken (1 1/3 pounds) as well as oil (2 tablespoons), miso, and scallions. Knead the mixture for about five minutes or until sticky and evenly mixed.

4. Wash your hands before coating with oil. Mold the mixture into 16 balls before pressing to form four-inch long cylinders.

5. Thread the meat cylinders onto the skewers, pressing lightly to flatten. Meanwhile, combine the basting sauce ingredients in a small bowl; strain and set aside the liquid.

6. Heat the gas grill on high. Cook the skewers for four minutes, turning them every minute, before brushing with basting sauce. Return to the grill and cook for an additional two minutes.

7. Brush again with the basting sauce and grill for the last time for two minutes.

8. Serve right away.

11 - Recipes For Treats

Claim your high energy levels back with these yummy, healthy, and added sugar-free treat recipes.

Yummy Nut Bars

Ingredients:

- Pistachios (1/2 cup)

- Vanilla bean extract (1 teaspoon)

- Pumpkin seeds (1/2 cup)

- Cinnamon (1/2 teaspoon)

- Chia seeds (4 tablespoons)

- Honey (1/2 cup)

- Almonds, raw (1/2 cup)

- Coconut, desiccated, unsweetened (1/2 cup)

- Sunflower seeds (1/2 cup)

- Lemon zest (2 tablespoons)

- Goji berries (1/2 cup)

- Coconut oil, melted (3 tablespoons)

Directions:

1. Set the oven at 350 degrees to preheat. Meanwhile, use parchment paper to line a brownie tin (9x9).

2. Place the nuts on a cutting board. Chop roughly and place in a large bowl. Add the remaining ingredients and toss to combine.

3. Transfer the nut mixture into the brownie tin, pressing down to form an even layer.

4. Place in the oven to bake for about twenty to twenty-five minutes or until done.

5. Allow the cooked nut mixture to cool completely before slicing into equal sized bars. Place in the refrigerator to chill for two hours or until extra firm.

6. Serve right away (or place in an airtight jar to keep for up to two to three days).

Coconut Vanilla Custard

Ingredients:

- Egg yolks (5 pieces)

- Vanilla bean paste (1 tablespoon)

- Nutmeg, ground (a pinch)

- Coconut milk (16 ounces)

- Honey (2 tablespoons)

- Strawberries (1/2 cup)

Directions:

1. Set the oven at 320 degrees to preheat.

2. Place the egg yolks in a large mixing bowl. Whisk well and set aside.

3. After shaking the coconut milk vigorously while still in the can, pour half of it into a separate bowl. Set a sieve (fine mesh) above the bowl.

4. Meanwhile, heat a large skillet on medium. Add the

remaining coconut milk and stir continuously until steaming.

5. Gradually add the warmed coconut milk to the egg yolk mixture, making sure to add it in a steady thin stream and to whisk as you go.

6. Add the vanilla bean paste and honey to the coconut-egg yolk mixture and whisk well until combined. Pour into the sieve-topped bowl containing the cold coconut milk. Remove the sieve and whisk until everything is evenly combined and smooth.

7. Transfer the mixture into small ramekins. Arrange the ramekins inside a casserole dish filled with enough hot water to cover the ramekins halfway.

8. Use foil to securely cover the dish. Place in the oven to bake for about thirty to forty-five minutes or until the custard has set, detached from the sides of the dish, and a bit wobbly.

9. Top the custard with ground nutmeg and strawberries.

10. Serve and enjoy.

Rich Coconut Brownies

Ingredients:

- Almond flour (1/4 cup)

- Coconut oil, melted (1 cup)

- Eggs (6 pieces)

- Coconut flour (3/4 cup)

- Cocoa powder (1 cup)

- Honey (3/4 cup)

- Vanilla bean paste (1 teaspoon)

Directions:

1. Set the oven at 320 degrees to preheat. Meanwhile, grease a brownie tin (9x9) with a little oil and then line with baking paper.

2. Place the coconut flour, almond flour, and cocoa powder in a large bowl. Stir to combine and set aside.

3. Place the eggs in another large bowl. Add the vanilla

bean paste, honey, and coconut oil. Whisk well to combine.

4. Pour the egg mixture into the flour mixture. Stir until evenly combined and smooth.

5. Pour the entire mixture into the prepped brownie tin. Place in the oven to bake for about thirty to forty minutes or until set and the center is cooked through.

6. Once done, remove from the oven and allow to cool completely.

7. Slice into equal sized brownies and serve.

8. Enjoy.

Coconut & Blueberry Muffins

Ingredients:

- Vanilla extract, pure (1 teaspoon)

- Coconut oil, melted (2 tablespoons)

- Baking powder (1/2 teaspoon)

- Eggs, large (3 pieces)

- Honey (3 tablespoons)

- Coconut flour (1/3 cup)

- Blueberries, fresh (1/2 cup)

Directions:

1. Set the oven at 350 degrees to preheat.

2. Use a bit of coconut oil to generously coat 6 muffin cups.

3. Fill a blender with all ingredients except the blueberries. Process until well-blended and smooth.

4. Add the blueberries and fold into the blended mixture.

5. Pour the prepared batter into the greased muffin cups.

6. Place in the oven to bake for about fourteen to sixteen minutes or until set and lightly browned.

7. Serve and enjoy.

Energizing Smoothie

Ingredients:

- Blueberries, frozen (1/2 cup)

- Green powder (1 scoop)

- Yogurt, plain (1/4 cup)

- Banana, frozen (1/2 piece)

- Milk, raw (1 cup)

- Protein powder (1 scoop)

- Avocado, frozen (1/2 piece)

- Coconut oil (1 tablespoon)

- Salt, Himalayan (1/4 tablespoon)

Directions:

1. Place the frozen blueberries, bananas, and avocado in the blender.

2. Add the plain yogurt, raw milk, coconut oil, protein powder, green powder, and Himalayan salt.

3. Process until the mixture is well-combined and smooth.

4. Serve immediately.

5. Enjoy.

12 - Lifestyle Changes to Complement the Adrenal Fatigue Diet

Exercise

Commit to moving every day - and having fun while you're at it – for any period of time you think suits you with your schedule and state of health. That might mean dancing for half an hour in an aerobics class, or performing slow yoga poses for five minutes.

The important thing is that you give yourself a chance to reach reasonable exercise goals while building a pattern of progress. Keep in mind that what you are aiming for is enjoying yourself and creating exercise habits; duration and intensity are things you will have to deal with later.

Consider different activities such as dancing in the bedroom, kickboxing to videos, power walking with your pet dog, climbing rock walls, stationary bike pedaling as you read a book, or taking ballroom dance classes, until you find several activities that you actually have fun doing.

Your body and adrenal glands will receive the greatest health benefit if you keep your workouts pleasurable and non-competitive. You will eventually find it easy to make time for exercise every day, and this can lead you to having more energy, feeling more satisfied, and experiencing a sense of well-being. It becomes much easier afterwards to exercise more intensely for longer.

Try tailoring your exercise level to what your body can cope with. This is an important thing you need to do to avoid compromising your adrenal glands' stress response system. Know that exercising intensely or working out for extended periods of time can cause your adrenal glands to respond more aggressively and get stressed.

Make sure to keep your workouts from becoming too grueling that they keep you from wanting to exercise ever again. Choose activities that make you feel good about yourself afterwards. During those days when you just don't feel like doing anything, try gradually easing yourself into your routine until you get the ball rolling.

On the other hand, on those days when you actually overdo it, cut back on the duration and intensity the next time, especially if the last workout you did only made you feel worse afterwards. Schedule a time to do your exercises. That way, you avoid putting it until the last minute, by which time you no longer want to work out.

Oxygen Intake

Practice correct breathing. Make sure to inhale through your nostrils - this promotes a slower but deeper pattern of breathing that is ideal for increasing your intake of oxygen. If you find it difficult at first to breathe through the nostrils, it is best to consciously breathe in slowly and deeply as often as you can. It also helps to see to it that your chest and abdomen are moving in unison as your breathe.

Try this simple breathing exercise one to two times daily for five to ten minutes. It has you breathing from deep within your belly, which promotes improved breathing efficiency and increased oxygen intake.

- Lie on the bed in the supine position, or sit upright on a chair.

- Cover your stomach with one hand, palm facing down. Do the same to your chest with the other hand.

- Gradually count from 1 to 4, making sure to feel the hand you placed on your stomach rise first as if a balloon is expanding inside.

- For a brief moment, hold your breath and then exhale while you slowly count from 1 to 4. Make sure to feel the hand covering your stomach fall first as if the balloon inside is gradually deflating.

Practice this exercise until you slowly increase the time you hold your breath.

Touch

Massages help your muscles unclench, your heart rate to beat at a slower pace, and your blood pressure levels to decrease. If your stress hormones have increased, a good rubdown from a pair of healing hands can help bring their numbers down. A quick or long massage has the ability to trigger your body's relaxation response as well as normalize your immune system.

Hugs from another person can help a lot in flooding your stressed body with the hormone oxytocin. This type of hormone is responsible for giving you a feeling of security and a sense of trust for that person. Oxytocin is known to help in reducing cortisol levels in your body, which in turn decreases the amount of stress placed on your adrenal glands.

Pets can have a calming effect on their owners. In fact, you will find that your stress levels are effectively reduced by the simple act of snuggling up to animals. Experience the comfort and calm provided by tickling your pet's tummy or scratching him behind the ears. Research has even shown how pet owners' blood pressure levels decrease when they touch their beloved pets.

Aromatherapy

Add several drops of essential oil to your shower floor to immerse your entire body with aromatherapeutic steam. You will experience a sense of your aura being cleansed as well as energized, which positively affects your mental and emotional state. Simply use a cloth to cover your shower drain; after several minutes, you can bask in and inhale the steam from the essential oil.

Make use of oil blends that nourish the body. You can pour about three teaspoons of your preferred carrier oil in a small dish, then add in about seven to eight drops of your favorite essential oil. Mix well and then apply to your entire body.

Just keep in mind that prior to doing this, it would be a good idea to do a skin patch test first. You can even use the same nourishing oil blend in massaging your hands and feet to help you feel relaxed all over. To give the scents enough time to blend synergistically, make sure to always pour the essential oil into the dish (or bottle) before adding the carrier oil.

Use a diffuser to fill your space with aromatic scent. Simply put twenty-five drops of essential oil inside a diffuser or a conventional oil burner that has a candle.

Consider **carrying your favorite scent** with you. Place several drops of essential oil onto your handkerchief or scarf (or even a regular cotton pad). Put the scented handkerchief or scarf in your purse, or place the fragrant cotton pad in your bra or pant pocket. The scent emitted will provide a calming/energizing effect on you the whole day.

During especially stressful days, simply **take a big whiff of your favorite essential oil**. You will find that this helps a lot in changing your focus and giving you a general sense of well-being. Try these scents: Lavender, rose, chamomile, ylang ylang, bergamot, lemon, rosewood, frankincense, marjoram, geranium, fennel, cinnamon, and vetiver.

Mindfulness

Mindfully eating your foods is an important part of your adrenal fatigue diet. You can practice mindful eating with these tips:

Eat your meal slowly

It would be helpful to spend five minutes concentrating on your food first, before you chat with the people at your table.

Take small bites of your food

This way, your mouth is not too full and you can taste your food more easily. You can place your utensils on the table between bites.

Chew your food well

This will help your taste buds detect the essence of your entire meal. Try chewing your each mouthful of food about twenty to forty times; you will be able to savor all the flavors in your food this way.

Allow all your five senses to come into play when eating your meals

As you cook, serve, and eat your food, make sure to pay attention to aroma, color, texture, taste, and even sounds made as it is prepared. Try determining the flavor of each ingredient as you chew.

Appreciate your food for the pleasure and health benefits it provides your body. Take time to really enjoy your meal as you eat it with friends and family.

Shop in a mindful way

Take time to think about the health value attached to each food item you write on your list as well as place inside your cart. This way, you avoid buying on impulse at the grocery store. Shopping mindfully also means avoiding the center aisles (where the processed foods are located) and keeping yourself from being tempted into buying the checkout counter's candies and chips.

Indulge in mindful resting

Take time to observe the sounds, tastes, sights, touches, and smells of things around you; acknowledge their existence and then forget all about them. It also helps to sit in silence as you concentrate on the way you are breathing, then allow your thoughts and ideas to come to you freely, after which you should let them go without you analyzing or judging them.

Try noticing any itching, tingling, or other body sensations from your head to toe, then let them go. And acknowledge your emotions for what they are, without planning to take any action as a response to those emotions. Accept their presence and then let them pass.

Other Tips

Write away your cares and troubles

Place a notebook and a pen on your bedside table. This way, you can write every little detail that comes into mind when you wake up. Write down all your thoughts about your financial dilemmas, job insecurities, failure to exercise regularly, or remorse over eating too much during dinner last night.

Make sure to include in your journal the things that you hope to accomplish in the next few days, weeks, or months. It also helps if you list down all the things you are thankful for. Then, tear up all those pages you have written down on and toss them into the trash bin.

Turn off your social media notifications

You will be surprised by how easy it is to feel less stressed once you take a break from the online world, and focus instead on living your life in "real time" terms.

Avoid alcohol during particularly stressful times

You would think that having a little alcohol to give you a temporary surge of energy and mood is worth it. But then you will be placing another burden to your adrenal glands, which will have to work overtime to keep your body in a homeostatic state.

Go outside and get yourself ten to fifteen minutes of direct sunlight

Sunlight boosts the release of serotonin, the brain chemical that is responsible for elevating your mood.

Refresh your mind by spending several minutes breathing in the outdoors' fresh air

This is a great way of clearing away those "gray" feelings you tend to have when you are under stress.

Give your mental energy a boost making use of

your imagination

You can start by gradually taking deep breaths as you close your eyes and visualize in your mind some pleasant thoughts or images. As you breathe out, imagine breathing out some unpleasant feeling, sound, color, or thought out of your body.

You can do this exercise for two minutes or until you observe your stress getting released from your body. Then open your eyes, breathe in deeply, stretch your muscles and go on with your daily activities feeling more energized and on a lighter mood. Repeat this exercise as often as you need; you will find that constant practice will give you quicker results in the long run.

Use acupuncture to stimulate your body points and give your body a boost of energy

With your index finger or thumb, press down firmly on an acupressure point and hold it for about thirty seconds to three minutes. Make sure to avoid rubbing the spot though; your aim is to simply apply a steady pressure.

Your energizing acupressure points include the spot over your upper lip, underneath the area between your nostrils, the spot on the back of your hand between your index finger and thumb, above your foot between the big toe and the second toe, and the outer part of your shin a few inches down your knee.

Try listening to upbeat songs to give your mood and energy an instant lift

In the morning, listen to happy, fast-tempo music while doing your tasks to kick your energy into gear. Then at the end of the day, listen to some slow music with a rhythmic beat to help ease your body into relaxation mode as well as let you regain mental clarity.

Laughter does wonders in stress relief

Hang images that tickle your funny bone in your workspace or at home. You can also watch funny movies or read comic books for an instant pick-me-up. Try laughing at your own mishaps and feel your tensions go away. It also helps to spend time with family and friends who know how to make laugh, and to whom you can share your own jokes and funny stories.

Supplements

Rhodiola rosea is an adaptogen herb known for being able to affect hormones such as norepinephrine, serotonin, and dopamine. Studies have demonstrated the ability of this plant to boost mental performance as well as improve fatigue, psychomotor function, physical fitness, and general well-being.

Indian ginseng (Ashwaganda) is another adaptogen herb that has the ability to reduce stress symptoms. It is also shown to produce calmness, which is why ashwaganda should be taken before going to sleep.

Holy basil leaf has been documented to be effective in relieving stress, protecting neurons, and enhancing mental performance.

Licorice appears to work for people who have inadequate cortisol in their system. Take licorice in the morning for a boost in cortisol production when you need it most.

Ginseng is a potent herb that has the ability to increase your resistance to stress as well as improve your mental performance. It also has antioxidant and antidepressant properties, as well as ability to naturally decrease blood sugar and blood pressure levels.

Astralagus root has immunity boosting properties that can buffer you against the harmful effects of stress. It does this by encouraging the production of more anti-stress compounds that your body uses to repair as well as prevent any stress-related negative effects. Astralagus root also appears to play a role in preventing cortisol from binding to stress receptors.

Thank You

As we reach the end of this book, I want to say thanks for reading this book.

I want to get this information out to as many people as possible. If you found this book helpful, I would greatly appreciate you leaving me a review. This helps others find the book as well.

This book was self-published with the amazing help of Self-Publishing Made Easy Now! [3] . You can grab a free copy of the checklist that started my journey here: FREE Self-Publishing Checklist [4] .

[3] https://selfpublishingmadeeasynow.com/xpjv
[4] https://selfpublishingmadeeasynow.com/free_checklist

Disclaimer

This document is geared towards providing exact and reliable information in regards to the topic and issue covered. The publication is sold on the idea that the publisher is not required to render an accounting, officially permitted, or otherwise, qualified services. If advice is necessary, legal, financial, medical or professional, a practiced individual in the profession should be ordered.

This information is not presented by a financial or medical practitioner and is for entertainment, educational and informational purposes only. The content is not intended as a substitute for professional medical advice, diagnosis, or treatment. Always seek the advice of your physician or other qualified health care provider with any questions you may have regarding a medical condition. Never disregard professional medical advice or delay in seeking it because of something you have read.

The information provided herein is stated to be truthful and consistent, in that any liability, in terms of inattention or otherwise, by any usage or abuse of any policies, processes, or directions contained within is the solitary and utter responsibility of the recipient reader. Under no circumstances

CPSIA information can be obtained
at www.ICGtesting.com
Printed in the USA
BVHW042016120423
662236BV00029B/520